Table o

Introduction

Doing Work That Matters

If we could all do just one thing in our lives, I think "doing work that matters" should be at the top of the list.

When we do work that matters, we have an impact on lives and make positive changes we never thought possible.

When I opened my private practice, my hope was that each day I could teach people to change the way they moved and impact how they felt, physically.

At the same time, I thought that keeping in contact with my patients even when they were not coming in for treatment was a good idea. Maybe an exercise here, or a quick tip there, so I could help even when they were not physically in the office.

So, I started writing to my list of patients. Since I opened the doors to my practice in 2015, I have emailed my list of current and past patients twice per week, no exceptions.

When my practice started, my list was short. First five, then seven, then ten people… and many times they would get read by maybe one person (thanks Mom!).

As the list has grown, so has the feedback to my writing, as in people are actually reading! Even better, people are getting value from it.

Each time I get a reply to an email, or a patient mentions they read my blog, I can't help but smile.

This book is a collection of writings that I have put together over the last few years.

Much of it is based on YOU - often, the questions and topics that come up in the treatment room, carry themes that I feel everyone needs to hear.

My hope is that this book makes you think… that 'common medical knowledge' may not always be THE best way.

If nothing else, I hope you enjoy reading this as much I have enjoyed writing it.

My Story

About once a year, I'll have a patient ask me about "my story" and why I do what I do. It's something that I have written about on my blog before, but I think it's worthwhile to elaborate where I have been in life, as my experience heavily influences my treatments, my interactions, and every decision I make within my practice.

In short, I both sympathize and empathize with every person that walks into my office because I have lived with severe pain & injury.

Here's the long version of the story ... As a senior in high school, I was on the Bridgewater-Raritan football team when, during a game, a player from the other team attempted to jump over me.

I guess he couldn't jump high enough because his knee dropped square into my lower back. Like any 17-year-old 'tuff guy' with a competitive spirit, I stayed out on the field and played for about two more quarters.

Finally, I was limping so badly that I had to come off the field and I collapsed in pain.

Our team doctor took me into the locker room and found blood in my urine. I went to the ER and they found that I had fractured two vertebrae in my back and also bruised my kidney (hence the blood).

I was released from the hospital the next day. So began the healing process.

At that time, the doctor said that I just needed rest and when the bones healed, I would be good as new... (If I only knew then, what I know now).

Six weeks later, I was cleared medically and after one day of practice, I was allowed back on the field to play in the state playoffs. It seemed odd to me that I could be in a back brace one day and the next, I was magically healed and ready to play a full-contact sport. But, what did I know? I was just a 17-year-old kid in high school.

Luckily, I managed to make it through the rest of the season, but over the next 5-7 years, I would get horrible back pain every few months. It would stay a few days and then go away and I remember that as soon as I would feel it coming on, I would go to the chiropractor. Each and every time, the faster I went in for treatment, the faster the pain would go away.

Still though, I had yet to address the root cause of my pain and I was merely chasing the symptoms over and over again.

This situation led to a much bigger problem a few years later and ultimately, to the reason why I do what I do today.

After high school, I went to college to play baseball. For the most part my back was healthy. Just a few times a year my lower back would act up and it would take a few days for me to recover. Then, I'd be "fine."

In my gut, I knew I wasn't fine. I had yet to get the care I needed and I thought about how many others might be in a painful cycle like me. I wanted to help others to get the care that I simply was not getting. So, I decided to enroll in chiropractic school.

And this is where the story gets really interesting.

One day, while playing basketball, I landed from jumping and felt an odd sensation in my leg. It was almost like an "aura" around my leg and I still can't really describe it. That night, I woke up with a burning sensation down my entire right leg. The next day, my hip felt like it was set on fire.

I sat in class for the first hour or so and when I stood up during a break, I had lost total control of my right hip, almost falling over.

Over the next week, there was numbness that traveled down my leg into my foot, until it finally settled on my big toe. At that point, I could not lift my big toe at all. I had lost full motor control.

As a student, I had the ability to become a patient in our student clinic and was taken under the care of an intern. Unfortunately, the treatment didn't do much – it neither helped nor hurt me.

I also sought out a Physical Therapist about an hour away from my school and began driving to see him every Friday. He was an expert in "McKenzie Diagnosis and Treatment," a methodology I use all the time in my office. However, it could not help me either.

I spent about 8-9 months trying all conservative measures but I was still enduring such bad bouts of lower back pain that I felt it was necessary to take the next step.

I went in for a surgical consult, and ultimately I had an L4-L5 Discectomy. Without too much detail, let me explain what this procedure does.

Think of your spine like a jelly donut and that a disc herniation causes the jelly to come out of the donut. And when you have a "Discectomy" you are taking away the portion of the jelly that comes out of that donut.

It took about two weeks post-op to be OK and at that point, I was back at school and treating patients full time.

Like the doctor I saw in high school, the surgeon recommended zero rehab other than walking.

I was far enough in school to realize that no post-op rehab was an insane idea if I ever wanted to be back to "normal." So, I began to write my own rehab program and became my own guinea pig. It was a true trial and error process.

I started out slowly lifting weights. Yes, weights. As I gained confidence and strength, I conservatively increased the weights I was lifting. With each increase, I would always wait until the next day to see how I felt.

Luckily, I kept feeling good and kept making progress until I was at full strength.

My "experiment" was the best education I could ever receive and went on to become a major part of how I treat all types of patients.

So, when I say to a patient "I understand," I really, really do. I understand what pain is like. I understand how it feels when everything you try doesn't work. I understand the frustration.

And most of all, I understand the fear that you'll never "be the same."

I beg my patients to understand the number one key to successful healing and recovery:

Take your time, and be very conservative.

Try every option before going for the surgical consult.

Surgery is great if it's actually needed. In my case, surgery was going to be there tomorrow or in 6 months.

Pain comes back if an injury isn't managed correctly.

Appreciate feeling good every day.

And remember, there is hope. You may think you are the only one, but someone else has likely dealt with something similar (e.g. me) and you can feel great again, just like I do now.

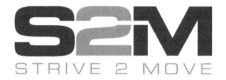

What Other People are Saying About Strive2Move

"He was able to get rid of my low back pain that had been persistent for a year, and just as importantly, helped me learn how to prevent any future injury. He made the experience very personalized to what I do on a daily basis."

-Brenda Hernandez from Basking Ridge, New Jersey

Do you want to experience the same results as Brenda?

Go to strive2move.com or call (908)547-0729 and apply for a 'Free Discovery Visit' to see how we can help!

Section 1: Fitness & Movement

Do You Need A Movement Coach?

The short answer is yes. Everyone needs a movement coach.

Why? And first, what the heck does that actually mean?

A movement coach may come in the form of a chiropractor, physical therapist, or strength coach. Truthfully, the title is least important.

<u>What's key is that this person is competent in assessing and correcting fundamental movement patterns.</u>

Some basic examples are the ability to squat and hinge with good mechanics and properly brace the core muscles.

Back to why everyone needs a movement coach ... Let's say you can't touch your toes. Or maybe, you have NEVER been able to do so.

Many people just accept a situation like this and say, "Yeah, I can't touch my toes." They leave it at that and think that's OK.

It's not OK.

You need to be able to touch your toes! Especially if you are like most of the people I deal with who are either active adults or athletes.

You see, things like a toe touch, getting your arms overhead pain free, and squatting are all motions we need to achieve and master.

This is where a movement coach comes into play. This expert will be able to assess you, prescribe exercise, and successfully enhance your movement so that it would be considered 'functional'.

Breaking or Bulletproofing You?

Someone emailed me the following question:

"… I'd really like to start working with a personal trainer but I'm just not sure who to choose. Do you have any advice or questions I should ask when going through this process?"

Many people arrive in my office simply due to the fact that they picked the wrong trainer/coach. In essence, they come to me to pick up the pieces of the 'wrong' that their trainer has done.

Imagine a situation where your knee or low back really starts to bother you. It's not that you just 'tweaked' it one time, it's that you loaded it with weight improperly, time and time again and now a problem has presented itself.

If your trainer is doing sound training, they would guide you to modify the workouts accordingly. This will make you resilient and resistant to injury. Injury prevention exercise is often just proper weight training.

Here are a few things to look for when picking a qualified trainer:

1. Do they have an assessment process? A good assessment process starts with a conversation. What are the goals of training? What is the injury history? What is the training history? The next step is a movement screen. A good coach/trainer will test things like shoulder motion, hamstring flexibility, and even the basic mechanics, like a squat or pushup, in order to get an idea of how best to start.

2. Who would they recommend if you have an injury? Having a working relationship with professionals who provide complementary therapies is a must! The fact is that even if they do the best training, they will have clients that have aches and pains and will need a chiropractor, PT, or massage therapist. **Caution:** some may try to 'play' doctor and give diagnoses to clients. If this happens, run away. Fast! The best trainers/coaches I work with are very quick to refer out and get another

opinion.Not surprisingly, they usually have higher levels of qualification than the trainers who don't refer out.

3. Can they see beyond fat loss? Most adults sign up for training to lose fat, which is a great goal. However, a good trainer/strength coach should help to see beyond the fat loss goal to help you build up strength and improve movement quality, thus reducing your chance for injury. Even if your goal is strictly fat loss, adding an injury into that equation takes you away from said goal. If you are in pain, you cannot exercise as frequently or as intensely as you would like…which makes you lose less fat in the end. Additionally, adding lean muscle through weight training will actually help burn more fat than strict cardiovascular training.

Doing What You Love Versus What You Need

Each year, I am afforded the opportunity to speak at a convention of Physician Assistants in New Jersey.

Whenever I present, I always leave time at the end for Q and A… and it seems that every year, I get the same question:

"What do you think of yoga?"

First, if you like yoga, I think you should do yoga. One of the main components of fitness is that you need to do things that you enjoy.

But, realize that if you really like yoga, you may need to do some form of resistance training as well. Yoga appeals to people who are very flexible because they excel at many of the yoga positions. And from my experience, people with a lot of flexibility (and who like yoga) often lack strength and stability.

Alternatively, think about a bulky weight lifter. He could do really well with some yoga training in order to get himself more flexible and mobile.

Fitness is first about doing what you enjoy. The next step is to figure out what you need. <u>Always make it a point to do what you love but make it a priority to do what you need.</u> If you always struggle with strength, sound weight training is important and if you struggle with flexibility, a routine of yoga or stretching would be ideal.

Does Your Body Have the E-Brake On?

"I need to stretch more!"

Many patients that I work with tell me this with a twinge of guilt … like the stretching police is building a case against them and they had better start soon!

Yes, some do need to stretch, while some don't.

If you have worked with me on any level you know two things:

1. Whether or not you need to stretch depends on a number of factors.

2. We are going to get you moving, assess you, and tell you the answer. As in, do you actually need to stretch?

Let's assume that you truly are tight and that some sort of stretching or mobility work is what you need.

The real question is "Why?"

The answer is NOT "because I'm tight!"

The real answer becomes more about what this tightness is doing to your movement patterns in everyday life, the gym, or during your sport.

The analogy that I use to explain it goes like this: "It's like you are driving down the highway, stepping on the accelerator, but keeping the E-brake on."

In this example, your car will still move. You will still be able to drive, but your engine will eventually blow out because it is working so hard.

This is just like your body.

Let's say you have really tight hamstrings and hip flexors and your movements are limited.

Now you go out to run and try to push it, hard. As you try to move faster, your engine will go but your muscles will hold you back.

You can guess what happens next: injury.

Having the right stability and mobility will give you the best possible shot to stay healthy over the long haul.

Section 1 Wrap Up:

My hope is that through this first section I have started to open your eyes to a new way of seeing your body and movement. Please read on for more insight and hopefully, more education.

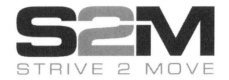

What Other People are Saying About Strive2Move

"Dr. Justin is fabulous! He listens to you and helps you to understand what you can do to help yourself feel better. If you want to work to improve yourself, feel better, perform better and be PAIN FREE, then visit Justin."

-Tracey Piparo from New Brunswick, New Jersey

Do you want to experience the same results as Tracey?

Go to strive2move.com or call (908)547-0729 and apply for a 'Free Discovery Visit' to see how we can help!

Section 2: Myths Your Doctor Told You

Myth #1: "Squatting is Bad for Your Knees."

Out of all the advice that doctors give, this one makes me laugh the most.

Patients often look confused when they come in with knee pain and say, "My doctor said squatting is bad for my knees." I generally smile at them because this advice is impractical at best, and downright stupid at worst.

And here's how the rest of conversation typically goes:

Me: "OK, Mrs. Jones, I hear what you are saying and I know that your doctor has the best intentions BUT can I ask you a question? How did you get from standing to seated in that chair? And how did you go from seated in your car to walking in to this office?"

The answer is usually silence. The point here is NOT to put down the doctor. It's to make everyone understand that context is important.

In other words, if the doctor meant that Mrs. Jones could no longer squat with a 400 lb barbell on her back, then maybe it is good advice. But, to never squat again? This is impossible.

Squatting is inevitable in our daily lives. What is most important however, is that we learn to do it properly and with a strategy that causes the least harm and discomfort. And just one more thing…Imagine using the bathroom without the ability to squat!!

Myth #2: "Never Lift Anything Over 35 lbs."

It's amazing how many people have told me that their doctor advised them not to lift anything over a certain weight.

My questions are always, "How the heck did they choose that weight in the first place?" Is it a formula they have? Is it that you may spontaneously combust if anything above that weight is ever lifted off the ground?

The truth is, we will all inevitably encounter moments where we need to lift a weight heavier than the subjective threshold the doctor set. Let's use that 35 lb limit as an example ...

This patient who was given that arbitrary 35 lb limit to lift has twins. I know that when they were little, she had to pick both up together. So should we tell her to never pick them up OR teach her a strategy to do so safely?

Everyday, even though we don't realize it, we will lift things that are heavier than we are 'supposed' to: grocery bags, shopping bags, children, furniture …

That is why I suggest that you do not shy away from lifting heavy weights. In fact, I believe you should make an effort to lift them. Often.

It is imperative that we learn how to do it with good form and proper technique so that we do not hurt ourselves.

Myth #3: "Walking is the Only Exercise You Need."

"My doctor told me I need to exercise and said that walking is all I need, about 30 minutes per day."

Many doctors are now encouraging their patients that exercise is important. This is a good thing! And much better than just doling out a prescription for the next 'miracle drug' that will cure all!

Yet their advice is problematic.

Walking – which is all they'll recommend - is simply not enough weight-bearing exercise to stop the inevitable muscle-wasting that unfortunately accompanies aging.

It's well established that we lose muscle as we age. This cannot be debated. Sure, walking is weight-bearing, but without using any sort of external force (resistance training) you are simply not stressing your muscles enough to maintain optimal muscle mass.

Logically, another question arises. How can we prevent muscle-wasting on our upper half if we never stress those muscles with weights?

We can't, and we won't.

An intelligently planned program of strength training and lifting weights is imperative for a healthy body at any age.

Myth #4: "If You Are in Pain, Just Rest Until You Get Better."

It drives me absolutely nuts when a patient comes to the office and says, "the doctor said I strained my back and I should take 4 weeks off from exercise."

First, this is such a defeatist attitude. In fact, I could make a very strong argument that 'resting' may cause more trouble. Yes, you may actually get worse!

The fact is that MOST people that are generally very active are used to movement and exercise. Simply taking all of it away does more harm than good. Four weeks later, they not only have an injury they're still nursing, but more stiffness and weakness from doing nothing for a month.

This turns into a vicious cycle that can lead to chronic pain for a long time.

My advice? Get advice ... from a professional who understands both pain/injury AND fitness to see if you can handle a modified exercise plan that allows you to stay active even while healing from an injury.

Take home: It's always best to try to work through your injuries with a sound and intelligent plan to get active and mobile again.

Myth #5: "Just Stretch It."

I have seen many people come to my office with a list of stretches their doctor gave them that should be making them better. But they still have pain, tightness, or weakness.

As you may have guessed, they just wasted 4 weeks of their life doing random stretches that did not improve their pain or function.

Here is a great tip:

If the stretching helps for about 30 minutes … and then the tightness returns, this should be your warning sign. Alarm bells should ring. STOP STRETCHING. Something else is likely going on.

If stretching was going to fix your problem, you'd already know it!

There are many reasons why your stretching may not be helping and most are quite complicated and confusing.

A quick example is an inflamed nerve. You feel tight so stretching seems like the best solution.

But if the nerve is irritated, stretching it will actually make you worse.

Take Home: Stop stretching if stretching doesn't take away or help diminish your problem. Something else might be the reason you feel tight and it's best to get to the true root cause!

Section 2 Wrap Up:

It's most important to me that you are not fearful or scared. I believe that true patient empowerment is first about busting common myths in the medical community that tend to scare the general public. I hope this section did just that for you.

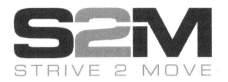

What Other People are Saying About Strive2Move

"It's nice, for a change, to actually meet a doctor who takes the time to really listen. How refreshing!! I have had to learn to allow my body time to repair itself by giving the exercises time to work, but results have shown me progress is possible. I also really appreciate the quick call backs when messages are left. Great patient- & customer-service!"

- Jodi Jacobs from Westfield, New Jersey

Do you want to experience the same results as Jodi?

Go to strive2move.com or call (908)547-0729 and apply for a 'Free Discovery Visit' to see how we can help!

Section 3: Managing Back Pain

Consulting With an Expert is the Best Thing You Can Do For Low Back Pain!

Many people come to me skeptical that I can do something to help with their low back pain.

I am proud to say that I very often can, even when they thought they had tried everything.

With technology these days, it's so easy to just search online and find good information on how to solve back pain by yourself.

However, what we say is this: "If information were the answer, we would all have 6-pack abs and be billionaires."

What this confirms is that information is not our biggest problem. Just because we can figure it out online, it does not mean we will learn how to do it.

I am a huge believer in hiring people who know more than me for help.

I personally pay a nutritionist to manage my nutrition and health. It's expensive and time consuming, yet I believe it's an essential part of my life. And yes, I know much of the same information that my nutritionist does, and I still see tons of value in making that trip to see him.

My hope is that Strive2Move is viewed as a valuable resource for patients.

And, even the ones who are knowledgeable about their body will still see the value in having someone like us in their corner.

Do You Always Find Yourself With a Backache Before Bed?

Have you ever gone through your day which included working out, picking up kids, and pushing heavy carts at the supermarket with virtually no pain?

But by the end of the night, after a full day of feeling great, your lower back suddenly gets worse and hurts?

I hear this all too often from patients.

I'm not surprised by it anymore, although I used to be. You see, most people would expect that their pain would be worse with all the activities they have to do throughout the day.

But in reality, what happens when you rest is as important as when you are active.

And what I mean is that simply finding a better position to rest at the end of the day could be an absolute game changer.

If you have a back ache that only comes on at the end of the day when you are trying to relax, your solution is to simply change the position you are relaxing in.

Pretty simple, right?

Let me explain further…

Most people at the end of the night end up in a position where they lay on a soft couch with their feet up on the table and put their spines in a rounded (forward bending) position.

It looks relaxing…except it is the worst thing you could do!

And here is why…

Flexing (bending forward) your low back for extended periods is by far the most likely cause for injury. And after a long day of being active, your spine is nice and loose and ready to be overstretched. It's prime time for injury!

Being aware of this is an absolute must. You are better off sitting upright with a few pillows as support or even lying down. Both positions will allow your spine to be neutral, healthy, and pain free.

Treating Through Teaching

One of THE primary tenants of Strive2Move and our 'Strive2Move Method' has nothing to do with our treatment techniques.

No, it's not about the manual work or the exercise prescription.

It's about teaching.

In fact, "doctor" means 'to teach' in Latin.

And it's important that we always remember this.

With that being said, I think it's really important to share conversations I have had that can be teaching moments for everyone.

So, I just spoke with a former patient who went to see a different doctor. The doctor took an x-ray of the neck and based on the x-ray gave this patient a diagnosis.

In this case, a diagnosis of 'radiculopathy' was given to this patient based on their x-ray.

The problem is that the diagnosis given simply cannot be seen on x-ray.

Unfortunately, this patient was given incorrect information. Yes, he could actually have a radiculopathy but it would not be seen with the x-ray study prescribed.

As I spoke with him, I could see in his demeanor that he was very concerned with the diagnosis or label that he was given.

The harm done is that now this patient has been falsely frightened into believing that something is really wrong with him.

Our goal at Strive2Move is to empower the patient ESPECIALLY when we cannot conclude that a diagnosis is 100% the cause of pain.

My advice: Always try and work with a provider or doctor who encourages you and does not scare you. Leave your appointment encouraged, not frightened.

How Your Back Pain is Just Like the 2008 Stock Market Crash

Who remembers back in 2008 when we had the worst stock market crash since the Great Depression?

It was so bad that at some point, people thought they may go to the ATM machine for cash and nothing would come out.

Very scary times, that's for sure.

But the question is this: What actually caused it to happen?

Answer: The mortgage bubble.

That's the easy answer, but I think most of you know and understand that it was way more complicated than that.

The point of this reference is that it wasn't JUST one mortgage that got us to the crash. No, it was thousands, if not millions of bad mortgages together that eventually made the bubble burst.

So, how does this relate to your back pain?

Almost all patients that come to our office with back pain will beat their heads into a wall attempting to remember the ONE THING that made their back hurt.

Of course, it's never just one thing.

Similar to the thousands of bad mortgages compounded over time, thousands of bad movements, poor postures, and tightness in certain muscles can cause your low back to crash or become painful.

I am always less concerned with the one event that gets the patient to my office. Rather, I am focused on the activity, jobs, and general movements that a person does everyday for 20-50 years that has put them in this precarious position of pain and discomfort.

Small changes, day after day will make or break you. A little good, done a lot, will help you feel great! A little bad, done a lot, will help you feel awful!

Making good decisions with our finances and our health over a period of time is what wins in the long run.

Remember, it's never just one bad mortgage or bad movement. It's always many over the course of time that puts you in a bad spot.

3 Reasons Why Your Back Pain Won't Go Away

One of the most common complaints I hear from friends and family is that they have gone to a chiropractor or physical therapist but that it did not work.

This often leads to a discussion in which I try to figure out the exact reason why.

After hearing this multiple times, I am convinced it generally has to do with three issues during the treatment process:

1. Excitement they are 'healed'- Most people are in a lot of pain when they seek treatment. As they start to feel better they also stop doing the things that got them there. Lower back pain is a classic example of this. Lower back pain just does not magically appear. It's months, if not years of bad positions and lifting habits that eventually cause the issue. The actual event where a person feels pain is just 'the straw that breaks the camel's back'. If a person like this gets lucky and feels better after only a few

days of treatment, it is natural to get excited and think they are healed. Again, not feeling pain is a horrible indicator of being better or healed.

The easiest way to illustrate this is with an extreme example. Let's say you got hit in the knee with a baseball bat. You have a huge bruise and a ton of pain. The doctor comes by and gives you some high dose painkillers. All of the sudden, you feel better but your knee is still bruised. You can see you still have tissue damage as indicated by the bruise, yet you feel fine. Again, this is a very easy example of pain being gone, yet the injury not being healed.

2. Consistency with care - We are all busy. I mean really, when is the last time you spoke to someone who said, "Yeah, I'm not busy at all." It never happens. Even with being busy, it's usually the people who are consistent with care that are the ones who get better and stay better. I see many people who start to gain real traction with their treatment and suddenly fall off. Many times, they lose

much of what they have gained and are frustrated as they need to start over.

3. Pain - I have heard of patients not coming in for treatment when they are 'in pain'. The first time I heard about this, I chuckled a little, thinking it was a one-time thing. However, now that I have heard it more than once, I understand it's a legitimate concern. Understand that if you have a flare up with pain, your doctor or therapist should be able to modify your treatment program in order to get you out of pain or at least decrease your pain. So, if you happen to be on a specific program that was working to increase your mobility, but you are now worried this program may make your pain worse, understand that so long as you communicate your concerns, a good practitioner should be able to make the necessary changes so that you get exactly what you need.

In conclusion, it's important to understand that we always have many factors that go into treatment. Whether it's one of the top three reasons I stated OR a different factor, it's important that the public is educated about this. An educated patient is always the best patient and the results will show!

Just Do The Opposite

As I further my career, I always try and take into account what I have learned and apply it. In some ways, what gaining experience in our careers becomes is simply pattern recognition.

As we experience something over and over, we learn that certain advice, or in my world, patterns, CAN solve the problems presented to us.

It seems that in my office the advice for injuries is that "doing the opposite" of whatever the patient has been doing is what works best.

Let me give you a few examples:

1. A patient walks in with lower back pain and a tight hamstring. This patient has been stretching his/her hamstring but finds that it only gives temporary relief. The way this person actually gets out of pain is by not bending forward and stretching the hamstring but my bending backward and stretching the lower back.

2. A patient has pain when sitting at his/her desk. The best way to break this pain

pattern is to do the opposite in which they stand up, walk around, and take a break from that seated position.

3. A patient who is very flexible has pain when doing yoga. Most times what they need is not more stretching or yoga. They need the opposite, strength training and stabilization. They need to get stronger by lifting weights so they can stabilize their body not by increasing flexibility.

In these specific examples, it is imperative to realize that the exercise and advice changes BUT the concept does not.

So think about this the next time your back is bothering you...

Are you doing too much of the same thing?

Would adding the opposite be the difference that makes the difference?

Section 3 Wrap Up:

With more than 80% of the population experiencing back pain at some point in their life, I think it is so important that we made this entire section specific to that subject.

Low back pain can be chronic and debilitating if not cared for and treated appropriately. Make sure you read and really understand as much as you can so you can avoid becoming a chronic part of that 80%.

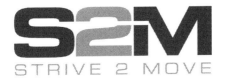

What Other People are Saying About Strive2Move

"My son was suffering from back pain and was referred to Dr. Justin by his football coach. We were told that he was the best person to help him and we couldn't agree more! He received excellent care and Dr. Justin was very thorough in assessing and treating the injury."

- Tami Kaetzal from Bridgewater, New Jersey

Do you want to experience the same results as Tami's son?

Go to strive2move.com or call (908)547-0729 and apply for a 'Free Discovery Visit' to see how we can help!

Section 4: Thoughts on Doctors & The Medical System

Why Your Dentist Should Not Be the Only One Doing Yearly Check-Ups

I am a big believer in health care, and not our model as it is today which would best be described as "sick care." Most of us only go to the doctor when we have a problem, not in order to prevent the problem from coming in the first place.

That being said, most chiropractors take a lot of heat for suggesting that patients continue to come to the clinic even after they are out of pain. To combat this notion, many chiropractors go on a public relations rampage and market themselves as "that chiropractor that only treats the patient until they are out of pain."

If you don't believe me, do a quick little google search on your local chiropractor and go to the "FAQ" section. One of the FAQ's is usually, "Once I am out of pain, do I still need to come in and get treated?"

The answer is usually something along the lines of, "No! Once you are out of pain, your treatment plan is finished."

The problem with this model is that it falls under the trap of "sick care."

For a dental practice, it would be just like a patient saying, "Hey Doc, my teeth feel good! I will call you when my cavity comes back."

In the world we live in today, we are conditioned to do at least our yearly cleaning or check up to make sure our teeth are healthy.

And we are also conditioned to see our regular doctor for a yearly check-up and blood work.

But who is the one checking your muscles, bones, joints, and movement patterns?

Just like many people get heart disease and chronic internal conditions as they age, they also get frail, lose balance, strength, and mobility, and suffer for years.

My advice is to be proactive about your health, including your teeth, heart, bones, muscles, and joints.

We each get one body, it's best to treat it right!

My Surgeon Said "I'm Good"

My surgeon said, "I'm good."

This is very often the conversation I have with friends and family a few months after they have had a surgical procedure on the bones, muscles, or joints.

Many times, the surgeon released them from care and gave them a clean bill of health. They feel great for a while, but in many instances a pain or ailment in that spot or elsewhere arises somewhere down the line.

In order to understand this concept, we must first really understand structure and function.

If we are talking ACL surgery, the structure (ACL) is what the surgeon works on. In other words, you have torn your ACL and the surgeon's job is to go inside and put it back into one piece.

What this means is that often times after the surgery, when the surgeon says, "You are good," what he really means is that his job is done because the ACL graft is solidly reconstructed back together.

But now, we must talk about 'function'. For most of you reading this, your function involves something more than just making sure the graft has been reconstructed properly. This means that if you still have very poor running or jumping mechanics that put your ACL at risk, the strength of the graft is only so important, as you still may be at a great risk for injury.

The important part is that we make sure you have function that matches your structural improvements.

To make life easy, answer this question:

Are you stronger than you were before the injury?

If not, your function is not where it needs to be. Make sure you seek a health professional who can truly get you back to the function you desire and deserve!

Which Doctor Should I Go See?

Often times, I have friends that reach out to me seeking medical advice for what seems like basic injuries (muscle pulls, low back pain, neck pain) and each time they are looking for advice only after going to their doctor.

Most often, they are frustrated because they left the office with a prescription for painkillers, an x-ray, and advice to rest. Intuitively they understand that this is not the solution they are looking for.

While I understand the frustration with the doctor, I think it's misguided. You see, our society has been trained to believe that any time something hurts, we must go to our primary care doctor. The problem is that with most of these type of injuries, the doctor can't really offer you much more than a prescription.

Please understand that context is also key. Just like you shouldn't come to me for a sore throat, you also may want to reconsider your primary care doctor for muscle, bone, or joint injuries.

Education is important. As a patient or healthcare consumer, the key is to know where to go with what type of injury or ailment.

I hope that resources like this book will leave the public more informed and therefore happier and more satisfied with their healthcare experience.

Is Your Doctor Asking the Right Questions?

I've always been told that I ask too many questions.
In fact, I admit it can be quite annoying.

At least now I am aware of this so before the barrage of questions begin, I preface by saying, "Sorry for all of the annoying questions," and then proceed to ask all of the annoying questions.

The good thing about my inquisitive nature is that it helps me do my job. In turn, it helps me help you.

You see, by me asking so many questions, your injury or your history begins to tell a story. Many times, you are not sure what the relevance is, but each question yields something that may be the key to solving your case.

-Pain in the morning or at night?
-Pain with walking vs sitting?
-Does stretching make it better?
-How do you feel after eating unhealthy foods?

-On a scale from 1-10 how much stress are you under right now?

The key is that the more questions we can accurately answer, the quicker we can usually solve your pain or dysfunction.

History taking and question asking is something that all medical providers learn during training. Unfortunately, circumstances often dictate that they question patients less and instead simply order more tests.

Be aware of this and make sure your doctor has time to talk!

The Problem with Specialty Medicine

Over the last decade, our medical model has moved from one of generalization to specialization.

This has caused a shift where instead of just going to a general doctor, you now go to the 'shoulder guy' or the 'knee guy'. This is great because since these doctors only focus on one thing, they are experts in that area.

You can fool them with almost nothing, except when the knee pain is caused by the hip. Or the shoulder pain is coming from the neck. The examples are endless and I see it each and every day in practice.

One of my mentors used to say it pretty bluntly, "Where you think it is, it ain't."

Our body is one giant compensation mechanism.

To put it more eloquently Karel Lewitt said, "He who only treats the site of pain is lost."

If you have a shoulder problem and nobody looks at your neck and middle back, it is an incomplete approach.

If you have a knee problem and they do not at least look at your hip and ankle, it is an incomplete approach.

Remember, everything works together and everything matters. As a patient, expect that your doctor checks and inspects more than just the area of complaint.

The bottom line is that specialists are great, when needed. However, taking a general approach to address the body as a unit is one that I believe is optimal.

I'm Getting Worse from Treatment, What Do I Do Now?

I am not afraid of making people worse.

I know, I know…nobody comes to me to get into more pain. And quite frankly, five years ago I would have never made this statement.

But as I have gained more experience, I realized that temporary increases in pain may not be the worst thing in the world.

In fact, I would argue that for something that is chronic or long standing, the results I want to see most are listed below in order of importance:

1. Improvement - This is obvious. I would love for people to improve immediately.

2. Get worse - This isn't so obvious but if I am tactical in my treatment methodology, I will know what caused it and that will give me great information moving forward.

3. No change - This means that whatever treatment I chose did not have enough of an impact for anything substantial to happen. I still do not have enough information.

Let me give you an example so that you can get a real idea of what I am talking about.

I often have people come in with suspected nerve irritation. It is tight, burning, and painful. What this person usually asks is, "Should I stretch it, foam roll it, or use a lacrosse ball to get the knot out?"

The truth: I'm not sure until I test it. So, if we want to know if rolling the area is helpful, I will do manual treatment on the area and see the result.

If it is true nerve irritation, they will probably get worse from this type of treatment. And when they do, I'm not upset because I just ruled out a possible treatment technique.

Furthermore, I probably saved this person from themselves. Do you know how many people are trying to massage an irritated nerve and wonder why they have not gotten any better?

Where many run into problems is when they get worse from treatment but the doctor or therapist uses a 'one size fits all' approach. In this approach, multiple treatment methodologies are administered by the treating doctor. And when the patient responds poorly there is no way to tell which approach made them worse.

Always work with someone with a specific plan of action. Do not be afraid to question them on what they are doing. If they don't have a good explanation or sound answer, you know it's time to find a new practitioner.

Section 4 Wrap Up:

I feel it is my job to not only treat pain but teach people how to be a more educated healthcare consumer.

In some cases, it is simply expectations and a lack of knowledge that leads people down the wrong path in regard to their health.

Be aware that simply seeking out the right care is more than half the battle.

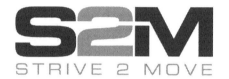

What Other People are Saying About Strive2Move

"I saw Dr. Justin when I woke up one day with severe back pain. Dr. Justin took time to evaluate me and walk me through what he was doing at every step. Once he spent approximately 45 minutes with me, he evaluated me again and also gave me exercises to complete at home so I did not have the same problem. I would recommend Dr. Justin to anyone!"

- Sean O'Brien from Bridgewater, New Jersey

Do you want to experience the same results as Sean?

Go to strive2move.com or call (908)547-0729 and apply for a 'Free Discovery Visit' to see how we can help!

Conclusion

Now that you have finished this book, I ask only one thing.

Help us do work that matters.

Share this book with someone you know who is suffering from pain, can't get back to their fitness routine, or wants to get back to doing what they love... even if another doctor told them they can't.

If you don't want to give up your copy, email me directly at drjustin@strive2move.com and I will send out a FREE copy to whomever asks.

If you aren't yet a patient at Strive2Move, and would still like to receive our emails, send me a personal email (drjustin@strive2move.com) and I will add you to the list.

For more free advice and information please go to our website at strive2move.com.

Thanks so much for reading!

Made in the USA
Columbia, SC
09 April 2018